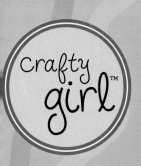

crafty girl™

W9-AJO-656

hair

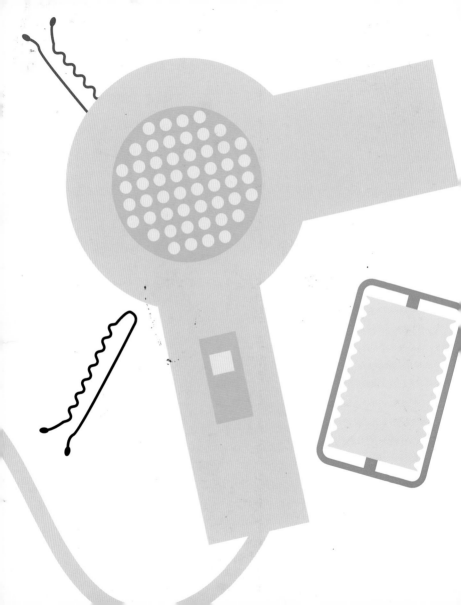

acknowledgments

Tangle-free thanks to Alain, Judy, and Victoria Traig.
Deep-conditioning gratitude to Leslie Davisson,
Mikyla Bruder, Gayle Chin and Stephanie Sadler, who
have great clever brains beneath their stylish 'dos.

table of contents

*L*et's begin by admitting that what's on top of your head is not nearly as important as what's inside it. Hair will not do your math homework for you. Hair cannot write or paint. Hair cannot run for president, although a really great cut *could* help get you elected. There's something magical about hair. It is an infinitely complex substance. Hair is encoded with as much information as a computer chip. It contains your DNA and absorbs what you absorb, revealing who you are and what you've been up to. A single hair can solve a crime. And sometimes hair itself is the crime (Mullets? Rattails? What were we thinking?).

All in all, though, hair is fun and fabulous and forgiving. It keeps your head warm and gives you something to twirl around your finger when you're bored. It's more versatile than Spam. It can be straightened or spiked, curled or crimped. The best part: Even if you go wrong, it grows out good as new. It's your crowning glory, and *Crafty Girl: Hair* is here to help you make the most of it.

Humans have been doing outrageous things to their hair from the dawn of time. Cave folk adorned their manes with bones. Ancient Goths artificially receded their hairlines by shaving them back. Sumerian girls powdered their 'dos with gold, and Elizabethan women dusted theirs with flour. In the eighteenth century, fashionable folks worked wire springs and horsehair into elaborate styles that sometimes attracted rodents. Go ahead and laugh, but some of the stuff we do is pretty crazy, too. Remember that time you tried to lighten your hair with butterscotch pudding? Enough said.

Well, not to worry. *Crafty Girl: Hair* has plenty of sane and sensible styling tips for you. Part 1, "Hair: An Owner's Manual," will walk you through all the beauty basics. Learn to navigate the shampoo aisle with our no-nonsense Product Primer (page 16). Tools of the Trade (page 21) will teach you how to use hardware like blow-dryers, curling irons, and crimpers. In Working with the Hair You Have (page 24), you'll learn how to tame the wild frizz-beast and wake up limp locks, to get great shine and body. You'll discover the secrets of switches, wigs, extensions, and color with Faking It (page 36). Finally, you'll learn how to banish bad hair days forever, thanks to Bad Hair Day Rx (page 37).

After you master the basics, put your skills to the test with the looks in "High-Style How-Tos." Practice the Ponytail Variations (page 46) or Farrah Feathers (page 55). Get fancy with a

Froufrou French Twist (page 57) or a Chi Chi Chignon (page 44). Get funky with Braidapalooza (page 42), Instant Gratification Dreadlocks (page 54), or Punk Princess Spikes (page 68). Time-travel with retro looks like the That Girl Flip (page 63) or the Veronica Lake Peekaboo 'Do (page 51). Or go bonkers, Bouffant Betty-style (page 60).

Once you've got your hair looking its best, it's time to gild the lily with some homemade hair ornaments. The crafts in "Hair Jewels" will help you do just that. Make Magic Floating Hair Sparklers (page 94) or Debutante Diamond Clips (page 79). Keep it pretty and natural with an Indian Princess Suede-Braid Headband (page 74) or a Tahiti-Sweetie Flower Clip (page 83). And if hair disaster should ever strike, whip up a Gypsy Fortune-Teller Kerchief (page 95) or a Kitty Cat Hat (page 98) to hide under.

Or instead of covering the root of the problem, craft a creamy concoction to fix that messy mane. The recipes in "Hair Potions" will restore your hair to shiny shipshape. Treat yourself to an Intensive Care Repair Mask (pages 109 and 110) or a Honey Hair Gloss (page 114). Indulge in a Lemon Soufflé Conditioner (page 108). Then add some spark with Sparkle Potion (page 118) or Rich & Radiant Color Rinses (page 116).

Ready? Then let's head out! Your first stop is the drugstore. Load up on good bargain basics like sprays and serums. If you're planning to do some advanced styling using hair pieces, color, or fancy combs, a beauty supply store is your next stop. Then hit a craft, fabric, or bead store next to pick up some materials to make the hair jewels of your dreams. And if your hair is just too unsightly to take outside, take heart: You probably have all the supplies you need to whip up a remedy in your kitchen cupboard.

We've got barrettes to bead and bangs to bouff, so let's get styling. What are you waiting for? The sun is shining, the humidity is a frizz-fighting 0 percent, and the forecast is for nothing but good hair days ahead.

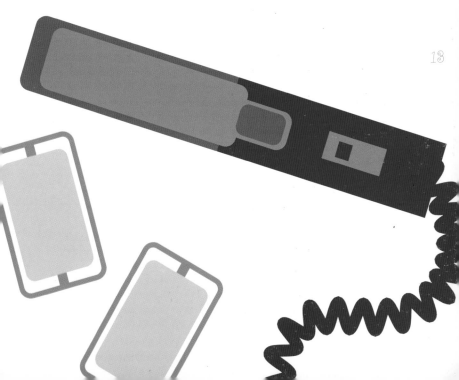

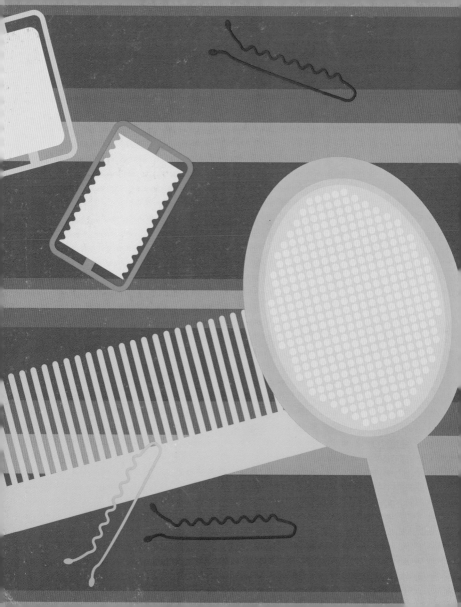

part 1

hair: an
owner's manual

product
primer

> Perfect hair in a bottle? We wish. Nothing can transform
> troublesome tresses into spun gold overnight, or banish
> bad hair days forever. But there are lots of products that
> can give you shine, bounce, and body. Here's a guide to
> what to buy, what to make, and when to use 'em.

The Basics

Shampoo

There's not much to say about shampoo. It cleans your hair
and that's about it, no matter how fancy or expensive the
brand, no matter what the label promises. That said, different shampoos do clean differently, so it's worth taking time
to choose the formula that suits you best. If you have dry
hair, pick a moisturizing formula and wash every other
day—or even less frequently, if you can stand it. If you have
normal hair, go with a gentle everyday formula and wash
every other day, or even every day, if you prefer and your
hair can take it. If your locks are oily, choose an oily-hair
formula and wash daily. Switch to a normal-hair formula if
your hair starts to get dried out. If you have thin hair, you
might consider a volumizing formula, which contains

ingredients that cause the hair shaft to swell. We've tried
these and haven't noticed any great difference, certainly
nothing like the ads promise, but on the other hand, it
can't hurt. On-the-go girls might prefer an all-in-one
formula, but be warned: these can leave hair limp.
Whichever product you choose, you should also use a
clarifying shampoo or the Clarifying Rinse (page 102) every
couple of weeks or so to get rid of product buildup.

Conditioner

We don't know what we'd do without conditioner. We can
live without food, water, and oxygen, but without conditioner we might frizz up into a tight little ball and blow
away. Conditioner smoothes out all the rough spots. There
can be, however, too much of a good thing, especially if
you have oily hair. Choose a light, everyday detangler and
be sure to rinse it out well. Normal hair calls for normal
conditioner. If your hair is dry or curly, use an extra-
moisturizing conditioner followed by a leave-in. If you
blow-dry every day, use a heat-activated formula to
minimize damage. And if your hair is really dry, or really
curly, consider using hand lotion. It sounds crazy, but
hairdressers swear by it.

Intensive Care Treatments

Hot oil treatments

Our very favorite hair potion. These always leave our hair soft and springy. If you have dry hair, get in the habit of using these on a regular basis. Save money by making your own (page 112).

Masks

If your hair has been replaced by a bundle of straw, you probably need a mask. Use a store-bought mask or make your own (page 109). You can make great masks from ordinary kitchen ingredients like bananas and avocado. If your hair is very dry, you may be tempted to try mayonnaise. Do not. We repeat, back away from the jar. We have the driest hair in the world and we tried this one time. We will never try it again. We had to wash it seven times in a row, no lie, to get it to look anything less than disgustingly greasy.

Repair packs

Repair packs provide an intensive infusion of nutrients and other conditioning agents. We've never had much luck with these. If you haven't been eating vitamins, we figure, you're not going to do a lot of good just glopping them on your hair. Still, repair packs have their fans. Experiment with a few different brands and see if you can find one you like.

Styling Products

Finishing Cream

Treat super-thirsty dry hair to a nice, rich, thick finishing cream like Alberto VO5 or John Frieda's Secret Weapon. This stuff replaces the natural oils dry hair lacks and smoothes out frizzies and flyaways. Regular old body lotion will do the trick, too.

Gel

The most versatile styling product there is, gel is a marvel of modern beauty engineering. It keeps hair smooth and controlled and lends body. Choose extra-hold for structured looks, flexible-hold for more natural ones.

Hairspray

The finishing touch. Hairspray is the enforcer—it keeps everything in place. Choose extra-hold for updos and structured or spiky styles, flexible-hold for more natural looks. Look for an alcohol-free formula if you use hairspray every day, or your hair can get dried out.

Mousse

A real '80s product, great if you're going for big '80s hair. It gives hair fullness and body. Because it contains a lot of alcohol, it can be drying, so it's not great for every day.

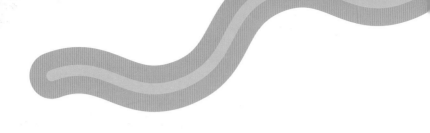

Polish, laminates, and serums

These silicone-based products coat the hair shaft to smooth the cuticle and add luster. They never seem to impart the glasslike shine we're expecting, but they do a pretty good job of taming rough spots and flyaways. Keep some on hand to treat hair tantrums.

Pomade

This is heavy stuff. When you use pomade, you're basically putting petroleum jelly in your hair. But sometimes that's exactly what you need. It helps short hair stick up and long hair stick together.

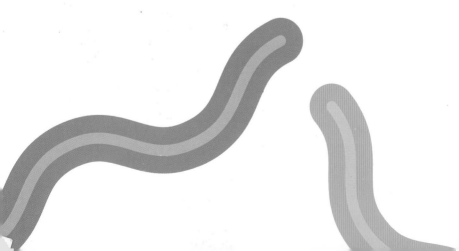

tools of the
trade

In the olden days, ladies had to style their hair with rags and red-hot irons. Happily, we've come a long way since then. Could space-age instant molecular hair-styling remote-control zappers be next? We hope. In the meantime, here's a guide to the modern hairstyling toolbox.

Combs

You definitely need a wide-toothed comb to comb your hair when it's wet; almost anything else will cause breakage. Depending on your styling needs, you may want a few other combs as well. If you do a lot of backcombing, you'll need a teasing comb, which features tines of varying lengths and a pointed end for lifting the ratted sections. If your curly hair tends to get matted, fluff it out with a pick comb, which looks sort of like a short-handled plastic fork with many wide-spaced tines.

Brushes

Your basic hairbrush, good for almost all hair types, will have soft, well-spaced bristles. Natural bristles are best, but plastic ones work fine, too. Depending on your styling needs, you may want to pick up some specialty brushes as well. If you're in the habit of straightening your naturally curly hair, a round, natural-bristle brush is a must. A flat paddle brush helps keep hair smooth.

Blow-dryer

Air-drying is best for your hair, but an on-the-go girl doesn't always have time. Blow-dryers get your hair dry and styled in a flash. If curl definition is a priority, get one with a diffuser attachment. If you use a blow-dryer every day, use a conditioner designed for heat styling to minimize damage.

Curling iron

We like to think of these as magic wands. Portable and easy to use, they give flat, limp, or out-of-control hair an instant pickup. Choose a curling iron with a small barrel if you're partial to ringlets, or with a large barrel if you just want waves.

Flat iron/Crimping iron

If stick-straight hair is your thing, a flat iron will make your life easier. For more versatility, look for one with a crimping attachment, for fun '80s zig-zaggy looks.

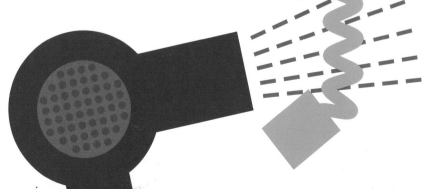

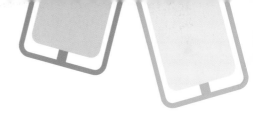

Curlers

There are all kinds of curlers, and one is sure to suit you. Old-fashioned pink foam curlers are cheap, almost comfortable enough to sleep on, and they provide some serious curl. Velcro curlers are convenient, especially for big waves, but can damage hair. Bendable stick curlers, another great option, are easy to use and effective.

Hot rollers

Super-fast and effective, these guys give great curl. The only downside: The heat can damage your hair, so they're not great for every day. Use a conditioner designed for heat styling to minimize damage. Better yet, use steam rollers—they're much gentler on hair, and the curl will last longer.

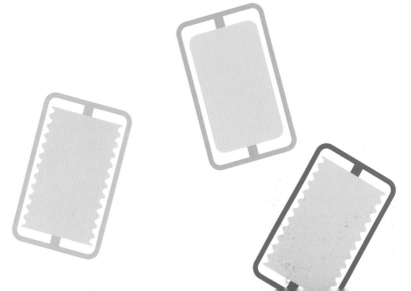

working with the

hair you have

The first step to great hair is determining what you're working with. Do you have wild red ringlets? Shiny raven flyaways? Amber waves of frizz? Every head needs a different kind of help. Here's a guide to what you've got and how to care for it.

24

Type

Dry hair

If you heat-style frequently, your hair is probably dry. If your hair is curly, it's probably dry. If your shoulders are covered with scalp flakes and your mane resembles straw, it's definitely dry. Don't fret. Dry hair just needs a little more TLC. Wash your hair as infrequently as you can stand—every two or three days at the most. Use a moisturizing shampoo and conditioner. Combat split ends with a leave-in conditioner. Avoid blow-dryers and curling irons, but if you can't help yourself, use heat-activated moisturizing products to minimize damage. Once a week or so, treat your tresses to a moisturizing mask or hot oil treatment.

Normal hair

If you can get away with pretty much anything, congratulations: You've got normal hair. Wash every other day, or every day if you prefer and your hair can take it, using a gentle everyday shampoo and conditioner. To keep your mane in shipshape, avoid products with a lot of alcohol and daily blow-drying, all of which can dry out your hair. When you need a little pick-me-up, try a repair pack or a mask.

Oily hair

You've got a lot of shine—sometimes too much. If you don't wash your hair every day, it looks limp and greasy. Not to worry. Acne is hard to control, but oily hair is easy. Wash your hair frequently. Use a shampoo formulated for normal hair, not oily hair—those can be too harsh. Go easy on the goop; no leave-ins for you. If you use conditioner, choose a very light one, formulated for oily hair. When your hair is looking extra-droopy, put a few good squirts of aloe vera gel in your normal shampoo and rinse well; that should perk it right up.

Texture

Straight

Your slick, sleek locks make you the envy of all. Blunt cuts and geometric 'dos showcase your sharp lines. The downside to being you: any cutting mistakes will show. So unless you've got a very sure hand, you'd best leave the trims to the professionals. When you get tired of looking so smooth all the time, you can mix things up by applying a curling balm and curling hair with hot rollers, curlers, or a curling iron. For just a little texture, braid wet hair and undo when it's dry. To combat static, use a solution of two parts liquid fabric softener and one part water as a finishing rinse. Or simply run a dryer sheet through dry locks. It sounds crazy, but it works.

Wavy

Your hair makes you Little Miss Versatility, and no one has more body than you. Wavy hair styles really well. Leave it as is, enhance the curl, or blow it straight. No matter what, it will look fantastic. To combat flyaways, use a silicone serum or laminating spray.

Curly

People can't keep their hands off your masses of crazy
corkscrew curls. The great thing about curly hair is that it
camouflages cutting mistakes; if it's uneven, it probably
won't show. The not-great thing about curly hair is frizz.
Keep things under control with an extra-strength silicone
serum. When you want a change, straighten your hair with
a blowout. Apply straightening balm to damp hair and blow-
dry, straightening 2-inch sections at a time by brushing
smooth with a round bristle brush.

Tight Curls

You've got gorgeous, over-the-top fullness and texture.
Embrace your wild ways. But if it's too tough to manage, a
relaxer can help. If you're not ready to make a chemical
commitment, you can relax hair temporarily by applying a
straightening balm and blowing it dry using a round bristle
brush, straightening 2-inch sections at a time. You've got
options. You can go natural and pick out a full 'fro, or you
can try something a little more elaborate. Tight curls hold
shapes well and are ideal for dreading or braiding. Your
hair is prone to dryness and breakage, especially if it's
chemically processed, so it needs extra TLC and gentle
treatment. Get a silk or satin pillowcase, or sleep with a
silk scarf over your head, to keep it from getting dried out
and damaged while you toss and turn at night. Frequent
hot oil treatments are a must.

getting the hair
you want

28

Choosing a Style

If you're itching for a change, your first step is to window-shop. What celebrity styles do you love? Which classmates have hair so cute it hurts your feelings? Flip through magazines, newspapers, even your yearbook. Try to get a picture of your anointed hair idol to bring to your hairdresser. As for finding the hairdresser, get a recommendation from a friend whose locks you like.

Next, you'll need to take your hair texture into account. If you have curly hair, think long and hard before getting bangs, unless you like looking like a poodle. If you've got stick-straight hair, approach layers carefully.

You'll also need to consider your personality and lifestyle. Sure, that feathered flip is adorable, but will you really set it every morning? Are you daring enough for dreads, or is a demure bob more your scene? How much hairstyling time do you have to spend? If you're an athlete, or just on the run all the time, fussy, time-consuming 'dos may not be for you.

Finally, you'll want to choose a cut that will flatter your features. Here's a quick rundown:

Oval face

You can get away with just about anything. Short, long, bangs, curls, layers—everything flatters your features.

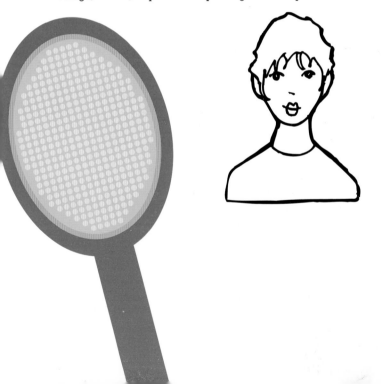

Round face

Avoid a baby-doll bob with bangs. A long, blunt cut is ideal, and fullness on top never hurts.

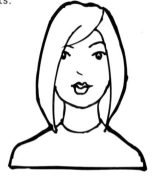

Heart-shaped face

Any cut that's full around that jawline should work.

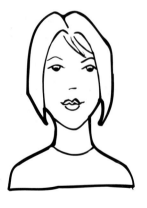

Long face

Go for layers around the face. Avoid long blunt cuts, and consider parting your hair on the side.

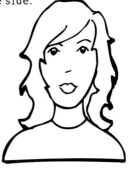

Square face

Long, layered hair is ideal for you. Avoid severe styles, like tight buns or chin-length geometric cuts.

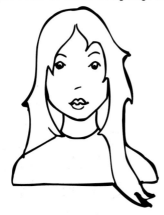

Chemical Processing

First, you should try to love your hair, no matter what. It keeps your head warm and gives you something to put barrettes in. Your hair is good. But if, after much consideration, you decide you would love your hair more if you could change its texture, you do have options. If it is stick-straight and you want to wake up with fluffy, bouncy curls, you can get a perm. The days of tiny-rod electrocuted poodle perms are, thankfully, over; today's body perms and spot perms add wave and fullness rather than frizz. Save yourself some heartache and get it done in a salon. If your hair is crazy-curly and you want it to be straight, you could get it thermally reconditioned. Thermal reconditioning is basically a reverse perm, and it really does work. Unfortunately, it's very, very, very expensive, and it doesn't work on African-American hair. But there is another option: chemical relaxing. Get it done in a salon or buy a very gentle no-lye at-home relaxing kit and have an adult help you. If you're planning on doing chemical straightening at home, don't attempt any color treatments; the combination of all those chemicals is very, very tough on the hair and should be avoided, or at least left to professionals.

Color

After "Hey Mom, check out my new tattoo!" the last sentence your parents want to hear is, "I'd like to dye my hair." Your parents have good reason to fear. Our teenage hair-color experiments did a number not just to our hair, but to the carpets and wallpaper. Dyeing is a messy business and you should think long and hard before you get yourself mixed up in it. Roots, fading, frying, split ends—it's a lot to take on. But rich reds, vibrant blondes, and deep blue-blacks can be hard to resist. If you simply must dye, and if your parents give the thumbs-up, follow this guide to getting the right stuff.

Temporary

Temporary hair color simply coats the hair. It doesn't contain ammonia or peroxide, so it's gentle and easy to use. It generally lasts about a week, and it's ideal for adding highlights. You can't use temporary color to lighten your hair, and if you're using it to darken your hair, be warned: It can stain light locks and last a lot longer than you expect it to. If you want something a little more subtle than that, try the quick color-enhancing rinses on page 116.

Semipermanent

Semipermanent hair color contains low amounts of ammonia and peroxide, giving your hair very noticeable color without doing a lot of damage. It's great for adding depth and richness, especially if you're into reds, but keep in mind that these often last much longer than the six weeks they promise, and if you're dyeing your hair darker, it may stay darker until it grows out. We learned the hard way that there's no such thing as "semipermanent" black hair dye, and whew, dealing with the roots is not pretty.

Permanent

Permanent hair color is the hard stuff. It contains ammonia and peroxide to strip your hair of its natural color and replace it with the new one. This is risky business, and you may want to leave it to the professionals. Be prepared to deal with roots and fading. Use permanent dye only if you really, really want big, big color, and you're prepared to deal with the upkeep.

Bleaching

There's no such thing as temporary bleach. If you're planning to go lighter, think really, really hard; maintenance is a major commitment. If you decide you simply must be a blonde, head straight for the salon. Bleaching hair is not a DIY activity. Too much can go wrong. Breakage, green tones . . . oh, it's too scary to contemplate. Leave it to a professional. And pick your professional carefully. Ask a friend whose color you covet for a recommendation. Finally, you may want to consider chunking, highlighting, or a weave instead. These techniques give you a nice blonde effect, but the upkeep is much easier.

Crazy Colors

If natural's not your thing, you can have a lot of fun with crazy colors. Most of this stuff is temporary or semi-permanent, containing little or no peroxide. They just coat or, in some cases, stain the hair shaft. So if you want a pure purple and blue or green, you'll have to bleach your natural color out first, which is a job best left to the professionals. But if you want to just overdye the hair you have, go for it. Be warned that some colors work better than others. If your hair is brown, green and blue dye will do nothing for you, but purples and magentas and reds will give you great groovy highlights. Blonde hair will absorb almost any shade, but may hang onto it a lot longer than the week or two this stuff is supposed to last. So if you dye your hair blue, don't be surprised if you look like a smurf until it grows out. Be prepared for the color to fade and turn as it washes out; black dye will turn greenish, and reds and purples will get pinkish.

Faking It: Fun with Wigs, Switches, and Extensions

You *can* transform your curly brown hair into straight blonde tresses, but it will take a lot of time and money and may result in a lot of split ends. Give your hair a break and head for the wig store instead. Wigs are a great solution for you instant-gratification, low-commitment types. Get a full 'do or a wiglet or switch. Wiglets are mini-wigs that you blend into your own hair to create the illusion of length and fullness. Switches are ponytails you can clip on and style—great for girls with short hair who sometimes envy long locks.

If you want long, thick hair by *tomorrow*, and you want to be able to swim with it, extensions are the way to go. Extensions are glued, braided, or wefted onto your natural hair and, if done properly, they'll look like the real thing. But they're not for everyone. They can be *very* expensive, and they need to be reattached every four months or so. If you still think they're for you, have them attached at a reputable salon that uses genuine human hair, and make up a good story to explain why your hair suddenly grew ten inches. Tell everyone you've been eating a lot of protein.

bad hair day

You eat right. You get plenty of sleep. You're kind to animals and children. You do everything right, and your karma is impeccable. But every once in a while, you wake up with a fright wig on your head. The bad hair day has struck again. It happens. We're here to help. Here are the most common symptoms and their solutions.

It's droopy, poopy, limp, and lackluster.

The problem is probably too much conditioner. Wash your hair with a clarifying shampoo and use a light detangler instead of a rich conditioner. Lay off the leave-ins.

It's poofy and parched.

Your hair is starving, and it needs the styling equivalent of a burger and fries. Grease it up with a nice, rich finishing cream. Regular old body lotion will do the trick, too.

It's pointing in all the wrong directions.

Afflicted with cowlicks? Not to worry. Just apply pomade or gel to the offending lock and smooth down with your fingers. Fix in place with hairspray.

It's just plain uncooperative.

Your hair may be too clean. Yes, hair can be too clean. Dirty it up a bit with gel, finishing cream, or a little light pomade.

It's frizzy as all get-out.

Does it sometimes look like a wild animal has taken up residence on your head? A frizz tamer will fix that. There are lots of effective frizz-control products out there. Choose one with silicone. Silicone is like a straitjacket for your hair; it'll keep your crazy locks under control.

Flakes!

Flakes can be caused by two conditions: dry scalp and dandruff. If your hair is dry and you've got little flakes, it's probably the former. A dry-scalp-formula shampoo and conditioner should help. Dandruff is a different condition altogether, believed to be caused by a fungus that produces bigger, clumpier flakes. It sounds gross, but it's not that bad, and it's easily treatable with dandruff shampoo. If the problem persists, consult a dermatologist.

Nothing is helping and you want to call in sick to school.

You've got a severe case, but it's not terminal. Trust us: It will look much better tomorrow. As for today, consider it an opportunity to show off your new kerchief (page 95) or a hat (page 98).

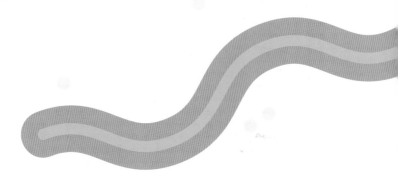

part 2

high-style how-tos

braidapalooza

You want green and blue streaks in your hair. Your parents want anything but. Here's the one hairstyle you'll agree on. Braid bright ribbons into your hair for a shot of instant crazy color. When crazy time is over, simply take them out.

You will need:

Pieces of yarn or ribbon, each cut to a length just slightly longer than your hair

Ponytail elastics

3-inch bits of yarn, ribbon, or fabric (optional)

[1] Grab a chunk of hair and divide it into 3 sections. Wrap one of the long pieces of yarn or ribbon around the whole length of one section, starting as close to the roots as you can get. Braid the three sections together. Tuck the top end of the ribbon into the braid as best you can, and secure the bottom of the braid with a ponytail elastic. If you like, you can conceal the elastic with a 3-inch bit of ribbon or yarn or Boy George–style fabric rags.

[2] Repeat until all your hair is braided. Or, if the all-over braid look isn't for you, just put in 1 or 2 braids and leave the rest of your hair down.

[3] Your amazing Technicolor tresses are all set. Now go out and turn some heads.

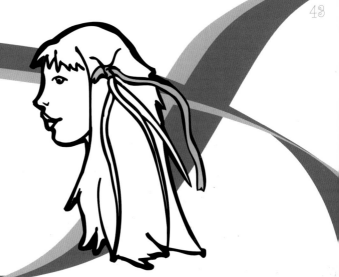

chignon

Chic and easy, the chignon is a classic for a reason. It looks good on everyone and it's always appropriate. It's also a great way to camouflage dirty hair. So if you've been too busy dashing from the museum to the ballet to hop in the shower, this is the fix for you. It's fast and fantastique.

44

You will need:

Shoulder-length or longer hair

Extra-hold gel

Ponytail elastic

12 or so hairpins or 2 hair sticks
(you could even use pencils)

Firm-hold hairspray

[1] Slick some gel through your hair to get everything nice and smooth.

[2] Using the ponytail elastic, gather your hair into a ponytail. Put it high on your head for a debutante effect, down low for a more sophisticated look, or smack in the middle for the classic version.

[3] If you like a braided chignon, braid your pony now. Otherwise, skip to the next step.

[4] Wrap your hair around and around the ponytail elastic, forming a bun (Figure A). Secure in place with hairpins or hair sticks (Figure B).

[5] Squirt on some hairspray for extra hold. *Voilà!* Instant sophistication.

Variation

Short-hair variation: If your hair is just a bit too short for the classic chignon, you have a couple of options. You can buy a fake one, and simply pin it over your pony. Or you can use a chignon form, which is a doughnut-shaped sponge you can wrap your hair around. Look for one at your local drugstore or beauty supply emporium.

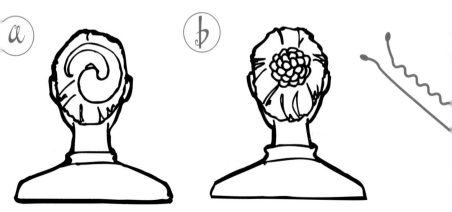

the ponytail
variations

Is any style more versatile than the pony? It can be preppy or punk, polished or pell-mell. It's easy and it doesn't require a lot of equipment. No wonder it's a favorite of both cheerleaders and heavy metal drummers. Here's how to achieve four of our favorite versions.

You will need:

Shoulder-length or longer hair

Medium-hold gel

Ponytail elastic

Bobby pin (for variations A, B, and C)

Crimping iron (for variation B, optional)

Curling iron (for variation D; a big one, with a 1-inch barrel, works best)

Chiffon scarf (for variation D)

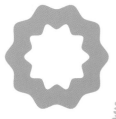

It's a Wrap (Variation A)

The pony at its most elegant.

[1] Slick some gel through your hair to get everything nice and smooth.

[2] Using the ponytail elastic, make a tidy pony at the base of your neck.

[3] Take a small section of hair and wrap it around the base of your ponytail, hiding the elastic. Secure the end with a bobby pin.

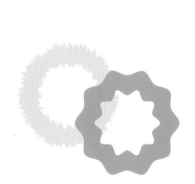
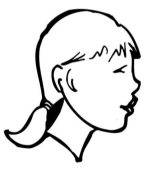

continued on next page

Valley Girl Side Pony (Variation B)

It's the classic '80s pony, and it's totally radical. Perfect for girls who just wanna have fun.

[1] Slick some gel through your hair to get everything nice and smooth.

[2] Using the ponytail elastic, make a pony on one side of your head, in the middle or a little higher.

[3] If you like, you can conceal the elastic by wrapping a small section of hair around it. Secure the end with a bobby pin.

[4] For the full '80s effect, crimp your pony with a crimping iron. And if you've got bangs, be sure to tease them up really, really high. Don't forget the giant plastic earrings!

48

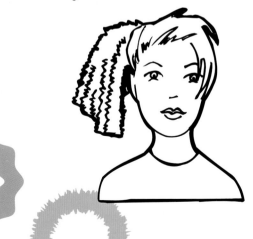

Genie (Variation C)

Your hairstyle wish has been granted. Now work that pony!

[1] Slick some gel through your hair to get everything nice and smooth.

[2] Using the ponytail elastic, make a pony high on your head.

[3] Take a small section of hair from your ponytail and braid it. Wrap the braid around the base of your ponytail. Secure the end with a bobby pin.

[4] Fold your arms and blink. It's hair magic!

49

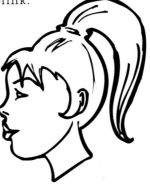

continued on next page

Girl Next Door (Variation D)

The classic bobby-soxer pony.

[1] Slick some gel through your hair to get everything nice and smooth.

[2] Using the ponytail elastic, make a pony in the middle of the back of your head.

[3] Using your curling iron, curl the pony to make big, loose curls. Curl small sections one at a time for the best effect.

50

[4] Tie a chiffon scarf around the base of your pony. That's it! You're ready to rock around the clock.

Variation Short-hair variation: Try a switch! See page 36 for switch tips.

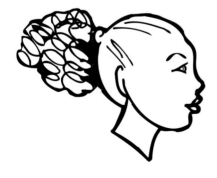

veronica lake
peekaboo 'do

Sure, it obscures your vision a bit, but who can resist a gorgeous, cascading waterfall of hair? In the '40s this look was so popular, and so dangerous, that employers banned it. Factory workers couldn't see what they were doing and kept getting their hair caught in the equipment. But as long as you don't plan on operating any heavy machinery, you should be just fine.

You will need:

Slightly dirty shoulder-length or longer hair (dirtyish hair styles better, so try not to wash it for a day or so)

Flexible-hold gel

Hairbrush

Curling iron (a big one, with a 1-inch barrel, works best)

Flexible-hold hairspray

[1] Slick some gel through your hair, then brush it until it's tidy and smooth. Part your hair far on the left.

continued on next page

[2] Take a small section of hair on the left and clamp it with the curling iron, clamp-side out, near the top. Pull the iron down the hair, smoothing as you go. When you're about 3 inches from the end, turn the curling iron under and hold for 20 seconds or so. You should end up with nice, gently curled-under ends. Repeat all the way around.

[3] Now you'll create your peekaboo curl. Take the front section of hair on the right side and twirl it around the curling iron, being sure to twirl in and not out (we want the hair to curl under, like Veronica Lake, not flip out, like Farrah Fawcett). Hold for 20 seconds or so. You should end up with a beautiful loose wave that conceals your right eye. You might have to curl it a couple of times to get it just right.

[4] Finish with a misting of flexible-hold hairspray.

[5] All set! You're ready for your close-up.

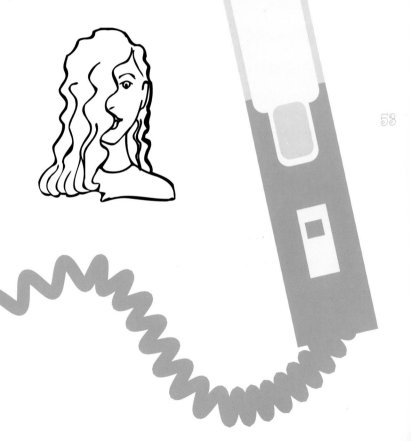

instant gratification
dreadlocks

Love the locks but dread the commitment? This temporary version will have you feelin' irie. Then, when you're ready to feel like your usual self, simply wash them out.

You will need:

Dry, messy, uncombed hair

Sticky stuff (use extra-extra-hold gel or spray starch; do NOT use a beeswax-based product, or you will end up with very, very permanent dreads)

Extra-hold hairspray

Lots of conditioner

[1] To begin, you will need a serious case of bed head. You get extra points if you skipped the conditioner the last time you washed your hair.

[2] To make a dread, take a small section of hair and douse it with your sticky stuff. Rub the section between your palms, twist it, and rattify just a bit by pushing the ends up towards the roots, until you've got yourself a little dread. Don't rat too much, or you'll never be able to get it out. Repeat until your entire head is covered with beautiful dreaded locks. Finish with a misting of extra-hold hairspray.

[3] To remove, wash your hair with lots and lots and lots of conditioner.

farrah
feathers

Next to disco, "The Farrah" was the best thing to come out of the '70s. This heavenly hairstyle features feathery wings that make you look like a well-coiffed angel, or at least a Charlie's Angel. Here's how to get your wings.

You will need:

Longish, layered hair

Medium-hold mousse or gel

Blow-dryer

Flat iron (a curling iron will also work)

Flexible-hold hairspray

[1] Start with damp hair. Slick through some mousse or gel, from roots to ends.

[2] Using the blow-dryer, blow your hair out. Turn your head upside down and really blast the roots for extra fullness. Part in the middle.

continued on next page

[3] Now, you'll make your wings. Clamp the flat iron or curling iron, barrel-side out, at the top of the front section of hair. Pull the iron down the hair, smoothing as you go. When you are 3 to 5 inches from the end, turn the iron out and slightly up. Hold for 20 seconds or so. Repeat on other side.

[4] Finish with a misting of hairspray for extra hold.

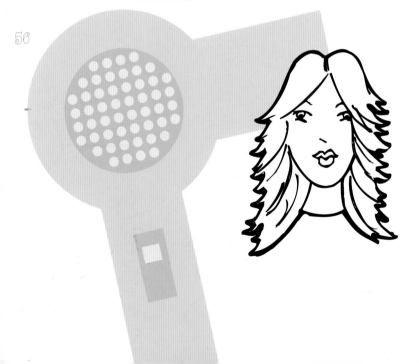

froufrou
french twist

French twists make us think of '50s movie stars: sleek, sophisticated, and mysterious. They can be a little tricky to master, but with practice and patience, you'll get there. Très jolie!

You will need:

Slightly dirty shoulder-length hair (dirtyish hair styles better, so try not to wash it for a day or so)

Extra-hold gel

Lots of bobby pins

Extra-hold hairspray

[1] Slick some gel through your hair to get everything nice and smooth.

continued on next page

[2] Gather all your hair together in a pony at the base of your neck. Don't use a ponytail elastic; just hold it with your hand. Twist the pony and turn it so the end is pointing up. Continue twisting until the pony coils and pulls into the rest of your hair, forming a hair "roll" (Figure A). This is your twist.

[3] Continue twisting until the roll feels nice and tight. If you don't want the ends sticking out, tuck them into the roll now. Secure with lots and lots of bobby pins. The pins should point upwards a bit, and should be close enough to the roll that they aren't visible (Figure B).

[4] Finish with a thorough misting of hairspray.

58

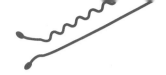

Variation Easy variation: Gather your hair in a low pony and twist. Turn the pony so the end is pointing up and secure it with a claw clip. That's it! This variation works great on shorter hair, too.

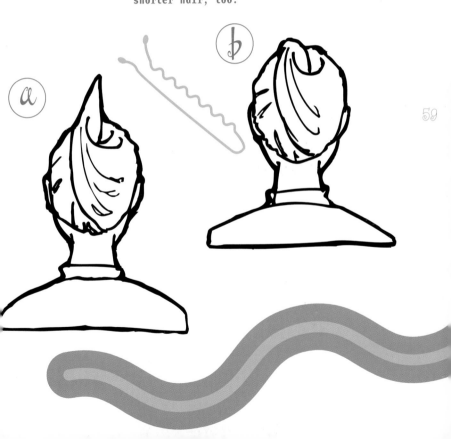

bouffant
betty

Known as "the Marge," "the beehive," and "the B-52," the bouffant is officially the most compelling hairstyle of all time. Equal parts intimidating and ridiculous, it is a hairstyle for the ages, fashionable as well as functional. It can double as a cobweb duster or even a coat rack. You cannot resist the bouff. Give in to the bouff!

Here's how to achieve the look yourself. We don't necessarily recommend you try it. It requires lots of backcombing, and it may damage your hair. But for some, a bouffant is worth a little breakage. We salute you.

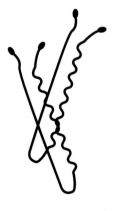

You will need:

Dirty shoulder-length hair (dirty hair teases much better than clean hair, so try to go a couple of days without washing it)

Teasing comb (see page 21)

Hairbrush

Lots of bobby pins

Curling iron (optional; a big one, with a 1-inch barrel, works best)

Extra-hold hairspray

[1] You'll begin by ratting the heck out of your hair. Ratting, also called teasing or backcombing, consists of combing your hair backwards, from the ends to the roots, to make a big old mess. Rat your hair section by section, until your head resembles a tumbleweed.

[2] Now you've got mass, but unfortunately, it's a mess. Next we'll try to whip it into shape. Using the brush, smooth the top layer of hair only, so it looks soft and silky, not scary and ratty.

[3] Using your hands and the comb, gently spin your now-smooth hair into a cone form. Pretend your hair is cotton candy. Secure the cone in place with lots and lots of bobby pins, hiding any loose ends underneath.

61

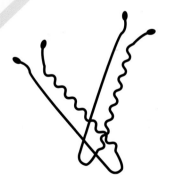

continued on next page

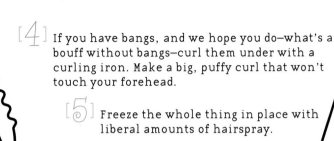

[4] If you have bangs, and we hope you do—what's a bouff without bangs—curl them under with a curling iron. Make a big, puffy curl that won't touch your forehead.

[5] Freeze the whole thing in place with liberal amounts of hairspray.

Variation Short-hair variation: Short hair can be bouffed, too. Instead of twisting your matted mess into a cone, curl small sections under, one by one, and pin in place. This is known as the "artichoke bouffant," and it's a delicious 'do indeed.

62

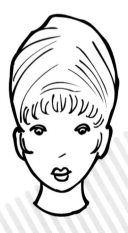

that girl
flip

Sported by Mary Tyler Moore, Marlo Thomas, and many more, the flip is the classic TV 'do. Perhaps it's because it's cute and kicky. Perhaps it's because it's so shellacked it can last through a dozen takes. We don't know why, but we know we love it. It looks good on anyone and it's easy to achieve. Who's that girl? One stylish lady.

You will need:

Slightly dirty shoulder-length hair
(dirtyish hair styles better, so try not
to wash it for a day or so)

Headband (optional)

Teasing comb (optional; see page 21)

Hairbrush

Curling iron (a big one, with a
1-inch barrel, works best)

Extra-hold hairspray

[1] If you want to adorn your flip with a swinging
'60s headband, put that on now.

continued on next page

[2] If you want a flip with a little height, you'll need to tease a little. Gently backcomb a few inches of hair at the crown (behind the headband, if using) by combing backwards, from ends to roots. Then, using the brush, smooth the top layer of hair only, so it looks soft and silky.

[3] Brush the rest of your hair to get it shiny and tangle-free.

[4] Clamp the curling iron, barrel-side out, at the top of a section of hair. Pull the iron down the hair, smoothing as you go but being careful not to deflate the mound you created with the teasing comb. Curl the ends up to make a flip. Repeat until you've got nice smooth hair with a good flip all the way around.

[5] Seal the whole thing with lots and lots of hairspray.

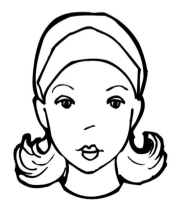

french braids

No one knows how to make a plain thing fancy better than the French. French vanilla, French toast, French roast— these are all great achievements. But the French braid is the greatest of all. Intricate looking but fairly easy to do, it's a marvel of hair engineering. It may take a little practice at first, but you'll get the hang of it in no time. A three-way mirror makes the job easier. Vive la France!

65

You will need:

Shoulder-length hair

Extra-hold gel

Comb (optional)

Ponytail elastic

Hairspray

[1] Slick some gel through your hair to get everything nice and smooth.

continued on next page

[2] Use the comb or your fingers to make a horizontal part along the "equator" of your head, from the top of one ear to the other. Gather all the hair from your ears up and divide it into 3 sections. Bring the left section over the center section, and then the right section over that. At this point the left and the right sections have traded their original places. You've started the braid.

[3] Take up a tiny section of the loose hair (below the "equator") on the left side of your head and add it to the left section of the braid (it will cross the center section). Bring the whole thing back over the center section. Then take up a tiny section of the loose hair on the right side of your head and add it to the right section of the braid (it will cross the left section). Bring the whole thing back over the left section.

[4] Continue in this fashion until there is no more loose hair left. Braid all the way down and secure with the ponytail elastic.

66

[5] Spritz the whole thing with hairspray for a little more hold.

Variation Easy variations: Once you've got the basic technique down, experiment with your own variations. You can tuck the braided tail underneath and secure with bobby pins. Try starting the braid at the base of your skull and working your way forward. Do two French braids, or even three. Or French braid the front of your hair and leave the rest loose. We're sure you'll come up with something new and fabulous.

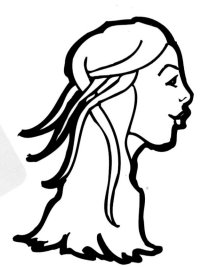

punk princess

spikes

Curly, girly looks aren't your thing. You like styles that come with a warning label. This spooky, spiky 'do is for you. Slick some extra-sticky stuff into your hair and sculpt the pointy, prickly hairstyle of your dreams. You can fashion a Mohawk, a Statue of Liberty 'do, a pincushion, or even a punk princess hair tiara. Sharp.

You will need:

Fairly short hair (you can make hair 5 inches long stand up, but anything over that is pushing it)

1 envelope unflavored gelatin (approximately 1 tablespoon)

¼ cup hot (not boiling) water

Extra-hold hairspray

[1] In a small bowl, combine the gelatin and water, mixing well. Wait a bit for the mixture to thicken and cool.

[2] When the mixture is cool enough to touch comfortably, slick it through your hair as you would gel.

[3] Shape your hair into whatever architectural construction strikes your fancy.

[4] Finish the whole thing off with a good dousing of hairspray for extra hold.

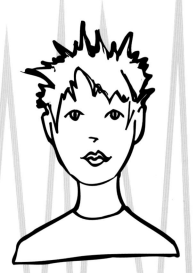

fancy-schmancy updo

> The prom is not about restraint. It's about glamour. It's about glitter. It's about a streaming, screaming fountain of hair. Here's how to achieve a fabulous forehead fountain of your own.

You will need:

Shoulder-length or longer hair

Extra-hold gel (make your own sparkly gel on page 118 for extra glitter)

Ponytail elastic

Curling iron (a big one, with a 1-inch barrel, works best)

Bobby pins

Extra-hold hairspray

[1] Slick some gel through your hair to get everything nice and smooth.

[2] Using the ponytail elastic, make a pony fairly high on the back of your head. If you like, you can leave a few tendrils loose in front to frame your face.

70

[3] Take a small section of hair from the ponytail and curl with the curling iron. Instead of shaking the curl loose when you unclamp the curling iron, keep the curl in an **O** shape and pin the **O** in place using a bobby pin, tucking the pin out of sight. Repeat, section by section, until the entire pony is curled and pinned.

[4] If you like, you can undo a few curls and let them spill down loose. If you've left some tendrils in front, curl those now.

[5] Freeze the whole thing in place with lots and lots of hairspray.

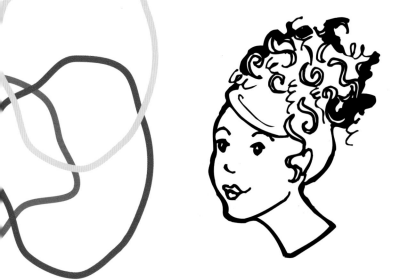

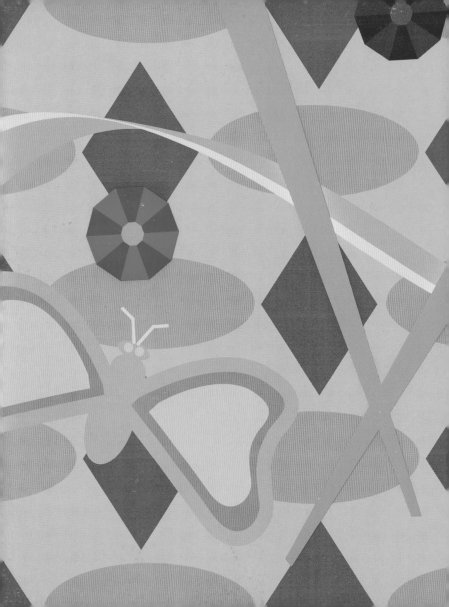

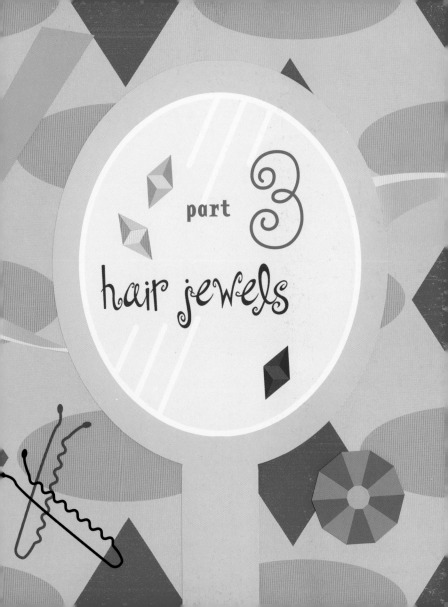

part 3

hair jewels

indian princess
suede-braid headban

This fabulous, fringey headband is the perfect accessory for casual country girls. It's neutral and natural. Pair with a denim skirt, cowboy boots, and a horse.

You will need:

3 yards suede cord (available at craft and fabric stores)

Scissors

Big chunky beads with holes big enough to accommodate the suede cord (optional; turquoise is especially nice)

 Cut the suede cord into 3 equal lengths.

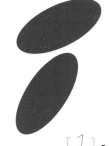

[2] Knot your 3 cords together, 4 inches from one end. Braid together, stopping 4 inches from the other end. Knot securely.

[3] If you like, you can slip a big chunky bead onto the end of each fringe and secure in place with a knot.

[4] To wear, just tie around your head, making a loose knot just below your ears. Be sure to leave the fantastic fringes in front.

butterfly
bijoux

We're not crazy about most bugs, but we love butterflies. They're dainty and colorful and enchanting. We just wish they weren't too skittish to wear as accessories. Since they are, we've made these beautiful barrettes from silk butterflies instead.

You will need:

Silk or feather butterflies with wire backing (available at craft stores, usually with the flower-arranging supplies)

Tiny flatback rhinestones and good craft glue, such as Aleene's Tacky Glue (optional)

Simple metal barrette

[1] If you want sparkly butterflies, glue some flatback rhinestones on them now. Allow the glue to dry.

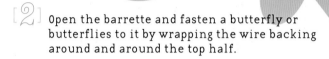

[2] Open the barrette and fasten a butterfly or
butterflies to it by wrapping the wire backing
around and around the top half.

[3] That's it! Clip in your hair and go mingle,
you social butterfly.

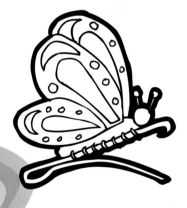

sweetheart
barrettes

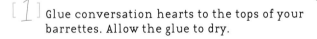

We adore conversation hearts. "LUV U" "BE MINE" "XOXO"—they're like candy poetry. They come in pretty pastels and go with everything. Glue some onto a plain barrette and you've got yourself a very lovable look. Cheap and easy to make, these are great Valentine's Day gifts.

You will need:

Good craft glue, such as Aleene's Tacky Glue

Conversation hearts

Plain, narrow metal barrettes

Glossy clear acrylic sealer

Foam brush

[1] Glue conversation hearts to the tops of your barrettes. Allow the glue to dry.

[2] Apply a coat of the glossy clear acrylic sealer to the tops and sides of the hearts with the foam brush. Allow to dry. If you like, you can add another coat or two for extra shine.

[3] Clip into your lovely locks and go out. Try not to break any hearts.

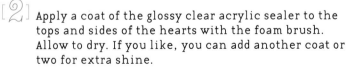

debutante

diamond clips

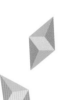

Plastic bauble barrettes aren't your thing. You're looking for sophisticated sparkle that's strictly top-drawer. These diamond-encrusted clips are dressy enough for a debut. Whip up a couple to wear the next time culture calls. Then start practicing your curtsy, because you'll be the belle of the ball.

You will need:

Good craft glue, such as Aleene's Tacky Glue

Tiny flatback rhinestones

Plain metal barrette

Toothpick

[1] Get your supplies and let good taste be your guide. Glue rhinestones to your barrette any way you like, using the toothpick to help you position them. Cover the entire thing, or glue on rhinestone polka dots or flowers, or other shapes.

[2] Allow the glue to dry.

[3] Clip into your shimmering 'do and watch your dance card fill up.

79

hippie-chick
beaded bobby pins

Do you have hair down to there? Shoulder length or longer? Here baby, there mama? Everywhere, daddy daddy? Then you need these groovy beaded bobby pins. They'll keep your flaxen waxen locks out of your eyes, and that's a beautiful thing. They look great in short, spunky 'dos, too. Peace.

You will need:

Bobby pins

Assorted beads (look for ones with holes big enough to accommodate a regular bobby pin, but not so big that the pin will bend; size-6 seed beads should be about right)

Good craft glue, such as Aleene's Tacky Glue

[1] This project is free and easy. Just thread your funky beads onto a bobby pin in any order you like.

[2] Apply glue to the last bead you thread on to secure. Allow the glue to dry.

[3] Make enough for the whole commune!

jeweled hairsticks

Avalon lives on in these richly jeweled hair ornaments. Fit for a queen, they're adorned with rubies, pearls, emeralds, and sapphires. (Okay, they're fakes, but we've got the royal alchemist working on it. In the meantime, make a set of these crown jewels for yourself.)

You will need:

Assorted fancy medium-size beads (choose sparkly crystals, pearls, semi-precious stones, or whatever you like)

2 head pins

Epoxy, like Krazy Glue

2 hair sticks (available at craft and bead stores; be sure they have a tiny hole drilled in the top)

81

[1] Thread a few beads onto a head pin, leaving about $1/4$ inch of the head pin unadorned at the pointed end.

[2] Apply epoxy to the top of the hairstick and the point of the beaded head pin. Insert the head pin into the tiny hole at the top of the hairstick. Allow the epoxy to set. Repeat with the other head pin and hairstick.

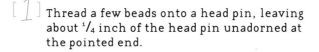

continued on next page

[3] Put your hair up in a medieval updo and secure with your queenly hairsticks.

[4] Command a loyal subject to bring you a mirror. Admire your fair hairsticks from all angles.

82

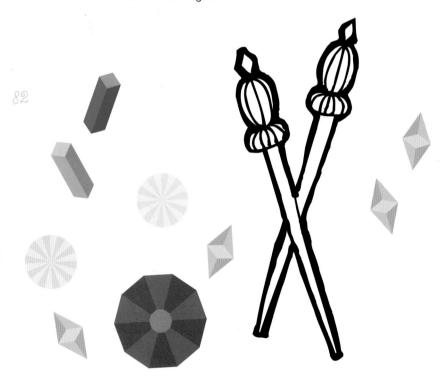

tahiti-sweetie

flower clip

Isle style is easy with this blossoming barrette. Accessorize
with a sarong, a tan, and a warm summer breeze.

You will need:

Silk flower with the stem cut off (the
bigger, the better; look for one with
a fairly flat back)

Plain barrette

Needle and thread

[1] Stitch your flower to your barrette. You
may want to sew it down at both ends of the
barrette to hold it in place. Knot securely
and snip away excess thread.

[2] Clip your blossom behind an ear,
or anywhere.

valley girl
retro ribbon-barrette

The '80s were not the best decade for hair. Mall 'dos, mullets—it wasn't a pretty time. But it did produce these rockin' ribbon-barrettes. They were all the rage in the '80s and they're due for a retro revival. Be the first in your valley to sport them. They're totally tubular.

You will need:

2 pieces of ⅛-inch-wide satin ribbon, each 1 yard long (experiment using contrasting colors!)

2-inch-long plain metal double-bar barrette

Good craft glue, such as Aleene's Tacky Glue (optional)

Teeny silk flowers or beads (optional)

[1] Holding the 2 pieces of ribbon lined up together, thread them through the open barrette, so they are under the double bar but on top of the clasp (Figure A). Center the barrette on the ribbon, with the loop end opposite the clasp end snug against the ribbon.

[2] Now braid the ribbon over the barrette: Take the ribbons on the right and bring them over the right-side bar and under the left-side bar (Figure B). Then take the ribbons on the left and bring them over the left-side bar and under the right-side bar (Figure C). Continue to the bottom of the barrette, tightening the ribbon as you go.

[3] Thread the last ribbon through so all the free ends end up on the same side, making ribbon streamers. If you like, you can secure the last stitch of the braid to the barrette with just a dab of glue in an inconspicuous spot.

[4] If your ribbon-barrettes aren't quite rockin' enough for you, embellish further by gluing teeny silk flowers or beads to the streamers. Allow the glue to dry.

85

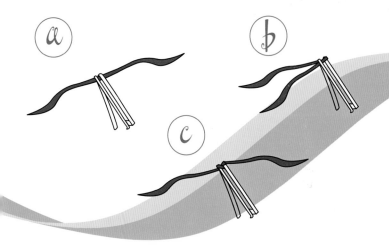

glamorama

boa headband

Big boa feathers in your hair isn't the look for everyone, but if you like over-the-top drama, this headband is the look for you. It's not a big production to make, either. Whip this fluffy confection up in minutes, then head right back out on the town. Fabulous, darling, fabulous!

86

You will need:

2 feet ¼-inch-wide elastic

10-inch piece of feather boa

Straight pins

Needle and thread

[1] Fold the elastic in half and knot the ends to form a closed loop, leaving about a 1-inch tail. Try it on around your head to make sure it's a good fit. If it's not, tie it again.

[2] Arrange the elastic loop in an oval, with the knot in the middle of one long side. Pin the boa to the elastic, centered on the side opposite the knot.

[3] Stitch the boa in place. Knot the thread securely and trim away excess thread. Remove the pins.

[4] Slip the headband onto your head and take your bows.

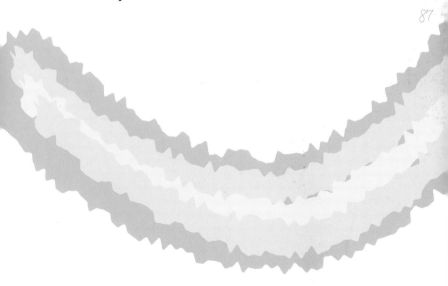

chopsticks

Sushi is the cutest food there is. It's so colorful and stylish, if it weren't for the smell of rotting tuna, we'd be tempted to wear it. Fortunately, there are odor-free miniature sushi erasers we can wear instead. Dressed up with sparkly crystals, they adorn these beautiful hair sticks. It's fashion, not fishion.

You will need:

Needle

2 miniature sushi erasers (available at cooler stationery stores and Japanese gift shops)

Assorted sparkly crystal beads

2 head pins

Epoxy, like Krazy Glue

2 black lacquer hair sticks (available at craft and bead stores; be sure they have a tiny hole drilled in the top)

[1] Using the needle, make a hole in the center of each sushi eraser.

[2] Thread a few sparkly crystal beads onto a head pin. Then thread on a sushi eraser, pushing the head pin through the hole you made in Step 1. There should be about 1/4 inch of the head pin sticking out of the bottom of the eraser.

[3] Apply epoxy to the top of the hair stick and the pointed end of the head pin. Insert the head pin into the tiny hole at the top of the hair stick. Allow the epoxy to set. Repeat with more beads, the other sushi eraser, and the other hair stick.

[4] Put your hair up in a chic chignon (page 44) and secure with your snazzy sushi chopsticks. Then take yourself out for some *tamago* to celebrate.

jeweled
headbands

Think of these stretchy, sparkly headbands as necklaces for your head. Make them out of pearls or crystals if you're fancy, turquoise or tiger's eye if you're earthy. They're so easy to make, you can whip up one to match your every outfit.

You will need:

Measuring tape

Elastic beading cord (available at craft and bead stores)

Scissors

Pretty pearl, cut-glass, or semiprecious beads with holes big enough to accommodate the elastic cord

Clear nail polish

[1] Measure around your head, placing the measuring tape where you want your headband to go. Cut a piece of elastic cord about 1¹⁄₂ inches longer than that measurement.

[2] Make a knot 1 inch from one end of the cord. Thread beads onto the cord. When you have 1 inch of cord left, make another knot.

[3] Tie the knotted ends together securely. Trim the ends and seal with the clear nail polish to prevent fraying.

fall-leaf
pony holder

This crisp, classic pony holder is the perfect back-to-school hair accessory. Pair with a plaid skirt and loafers and you'll get an A+ for style.

You will need:

Two 5-by-5-inch squares of felt in contrasting colors (dark green and light green are especially nice, but you can choose any colors you like)

Scissors

Good craft glue, such as Aleene's Tacky Glue

Embroidery scissors (optional)

5-inch dowel with one pointed end (a pencil is perfect, and perfect for back-to-school; choose a colored pencil that matches your felt)

[1] Take one square of felt and cut out a leaf shape approximately 4 inches long and 2½ inches wide. Glue the leaf to the other piece of felt, centering it in the square. Allow the glue to dry

[2] When dry, cut out around the leaf, following the contours of the shape and leaving a contrasting border all around it.

[3] Make 2 small holes in your two-layer felt leaf, about 1 inch in from each end. Embroidery scissors might make this job easier. Better yet, ask an adult to do it.

[4] To wear, gather your hair in a loose, low pony and top with your felt fall leaf. Secure by pushing the dowel through the holes.

sparklers & spookers

Affix rhinestones or pearls to Velcro backing for gems
that float magically in your hair like snowflakes. If you
prefer spooky to sparkly, affix tiny plastic bugs instead.
And if you like both, go ahead and mix it up, or glue a
few jewels to the critters.

94

You will need:

Flatback rhinestones, pearls, and/or
tiny plastic insects

Tiny adhesive-backed Velcro circles
(available at craft stores, fabric stores,
even hardware and drugstores; you
probably want the smallest ones you
can find)

Good craft glue, such as Aleene's
Tacky Glue (optional)

[1] Affix your gems or insects to the adhesive side
of the Velcro circles. You want to use the
prickly Velcro circle as opposed to the fuzzy
Velcro circle. If the beads and bugs don't stick
to the Velcro adhesive as well as you like, use a
little glue. Allow the glue to dry.

[2] To wear, simply stick gems wherever you
want them rubbing lightly against hair. The
Velcro keeps them in place. Be warned that
your gems might fall out later in the day, so
don't use diamonds.

gypsy fortune-teller
kerchief

We're not sure why fortune-tellers all wear head scarves. Maybe it's because they can see the fashion future. Or maybe it's just because they know it's going to rain. Whatever the reason, we love their beaded, bohemian kerchiefs. Whip one up for yourself. We see a stylish new accessory in your future.

You will need:

Simple, solid scarf (choose chiffon, velvet, silk, or anything you like)

Any or all of the following:

Assorted beads (seed beads and pearls are especially nice)

Needle and thread

Rickrack, ribbon, or trim

Embroidery thread

Embroidery needle

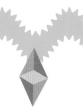

continued on next page

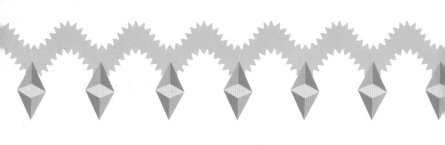

[1] Gypsy kerchief decorating has no rules; just get your goods and go for it. Stitch on a border of little seed beads or pearl polka dots. Make tiny seed-bead flowers. Sew on rickrack, ribbon, or trim. Embellish with embroidery. Stitch on vines, flowers, or whatever you like. When you're done, knot all thread ends securely and trim away the excess thread.

[2] Tie your new kerchief over your unruly gypsy mane and go find your future.

hair band

This simple hair ornament is a work of art. The ponytail elastic concept is reborn with beautiful velvet or satin ribbons to keep your Renaissance ringlets off your pretty-as-a-portrait face. Whip one up and wait for someone to write you an ode.

You will need:

Two 16-inch pieces ¼-inch-wide velvet or satin ribbon

Clear nail polish

Straight pins

4 inches ¼-inch-wide elastic

Needle and thread

Scissors

[1] Brush the ends of each piece of ribbon with the clear nail polish to prevent fraying. Allow to dry.

[2] Pin the ribbons to the elastic. Angle the ribbon ends a bit so they won't overlap on your head.

[3] Stitch the ribbon in place with needle and thread. Knot the thread securely and trim away excess thread.

kitty cat
hat

Cats have it so easy. They never have bad hair days.
Their coats always look great and the only styling product
they need is their own saliva. Okay, maybe they don't
have it so great. But you can still steal fabulous kitty style.
Hide under this adorable hat the next time your own lion's
mane won't behave. It's the cat's meow.

You will need:

Scrap of fleece (a 2½-by-5-inch
piece should about do it)

Scissors

Needle and thread

Straight pins

Store-bought plain fleece hat

[1] Cut four identical triangles out of your
scrap of fleece, each approximately 2¹/₂
inches by 2¹/₂ inches by 3 inches.

[2] Sew two of the triangles together, right sides facing, along both of the 2½-inch sides, leaving a ¼-inch seam allowance. Knot the thread securely and trim away excess thread. Leave the 3-inch side open. Turn inside out. Repeat with the other two triangles. Now you have your kitty ears.

[3] Pin the ears in place on your fleece hat with the raw edges of the ears turned under (the seam allowance should be about ¼ inch). Stitch down to secure. Try to make the stitches as inconspicuous as possible. Knot securely and trim away excess thread.

[4] Try on your new hat and go take a well-deserved catnap.

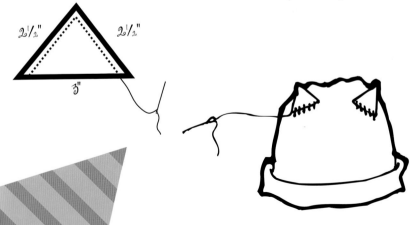

2½"   2½"

3"

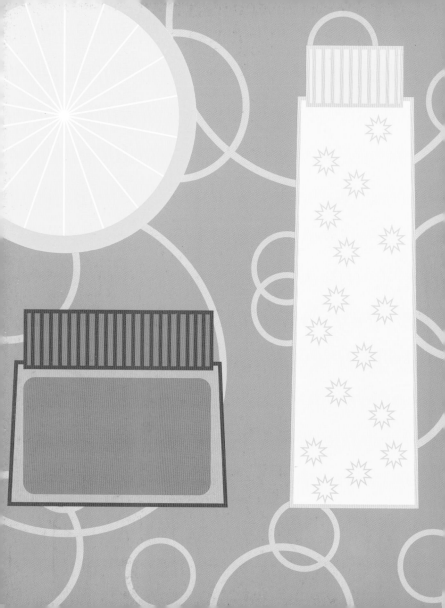

part 4

hair potions

Is your hair feeling funky and gunky? Dull and drab? Sounds like a case of product buildup. This super-sudsy shampoo formula will wash away the nasty residue and restore your hair's natural sparkle. Follow with the Clarifying Rinse for extra shine and softness.

You will need for Squeaky-Clean Shampoo:

2 teaspoons baking soda

12 ounces liquid castile soap or shampoo (skip the conditioning formulas, which cling to hair; clarifying shampoos and baby shampoos work best)

You will need for Clarifying Rinse:

1 cup distilled water

½ cup lemon juice (for blondes) or apple cider vinegar (for everyone else)

[1] Mix the baking soda into the shampoo. Apply 1 or 2 tablespoons to wet hair, working through well. Rinse out and condition as usual.

[2] For extra shine, combine the distilled water and lemon juice or vinegar, and pour over hair. Rinse well. Dry and style as usual.

Makes 12 ounces shampoo and one clarifying rinse treatment.

wildflower

shampoo

We just love fresh flowers in our hair, but they're not really practical for everyday wear. They wilt and droop, they attract bees, and you tend to get funny looks in the grocery store when you've got a rosebush parked on your head. That's why we love this floral conditioning concoction: It's got all of nature's goodness with none of the branches and bugs. It's shampoo with flower power and we think you'll like it, too.

You will need:

½ cup water

4 to 6 tablespoons dried wildflowers and herbs (available at your local herb or health-food store; choose sage or marigold for oily hair, rosemary or chamomile for dry hair, nettle for thin hair, or lavender for normal hair)

1 cup gentle, unscented shampoo (baby shampoo is best)

Clean, dry bottle

[1] In a small saucepan, combine the water and dried flowers or herbs. Bring to a boil, then remove from the heat. Allow to steep until cool. Strain and save the infused water.

[2] Combine the infused water and shampoo in the bottle and shake to mix well.

[3] To use, apply 1 or 2 tablespoons to wet hair, working through well. Rinse out and condition as usual. If you don't plan to use the shampoo within a week, store it in the refrigerator. It doesn't contain preservatives, so it can go bad.

Makes about 12 ounces.

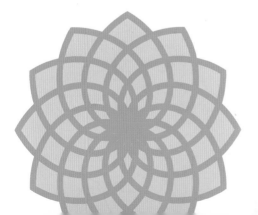

creamy coconut
conditioner

Give yourself the tropical treatment with this creamy, dreamy conditioner. It's as rich as a slice of coconut pie and much more nourishing. It's a little heavy, so it's best for girls with dry hair.

You will need:

1 egg

2 tablespoons coconut milk

1 tablespoon honey (optional)

2 tablespoons oil (any kind of vegetable oil is fine; if you want to get really fancy, use coconut oil or sweet almond oil)

[1] Combine all the ingredients in a blender and mix on low for half a minute or so. If you don't have a blender, you can use an egg beater instead. And if you don't have an egg beater, you can just use a spoon and a lot of elbow grease. (The mixture will smell great, but it tastes awful, so don't even try to eat it. Besides, raw egg is bad for you.)

[2] Take the coconut conditioner into the shower with you. Shampoo as usual, then apply the conditioner and leave on as long as you can stand it.

[3] Rinse out and dry and style as usual. Toss any remaining conditioner—it won't keep.

Makes one treatment.

lemon soufflé
conditioner

> This light, creamy conditioner is like dessert for your hair.
> It makes a great last course to your beauty regime, leaving
> you with a shiny finish. It won't weigh hair down, so it's
> ideal for limp or oily locks.

You will need:

1 envelope unflavored gelatin
(approximately 1 tablespoon)

1 teaspoon honey (optional)

3 tablespoons warm water

2 tablespoons lemon juice

1 egg

[1] In a small bowl, combine the gelatin, honey (if using),
and warm water, stirring until the gelatin is dissolved.
Add the lemon juice and egg and mix well. (The mixture will smell great, but it tastes awful, so don't even
try to eat it. Besides, raw egg is bad for you.)

[2] Like a soufflé, this mixture must be consumed right
away. Apply to wet, freshly washed hair and leave on
3 minutes or even longer. Rinse out. If there's any conditioner left over, go ahead and toss it; it won't keep.

Makes one treatment.

repair masks

Your hair is dried, fried, and you just want to hide. You need a mask. These yummy conditioning masks will cheer up your sad locks in a snap. You probably have all the supplies you need in your refrigerator already. So go whip one up right now. You and your hair will feel much better.

Banana Mask

This is a good basic mask, suitable for all hair types. You'll smell like a fruit salad, but who doesn't like fruit salad?

You will need:

1 ripe banana

1 tablespoon plain yogurt

1 tablespoon oil (omit if your hair is oily)

¼ teaspoon honey

[1] In a bowl, mash the banana. Add the yogurt, oil (if using), and honey and mix well.

continued on next page

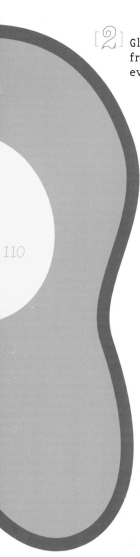

[2] Glop this slop all over your hair, distributing well from roots to ends. Leave on for 15 minutes or even longer if you can stand it.

[3] Rinse out and shampoo and condition as usual. Toss any remaining mask—it won't keep.

Makes one treatment.

Avocado Mask

This moisturizing formula is great for dry hair. Rich and satisfying, it's basically guacamole for your head. If you're hungry, mix up a little extra for your mouth. Bust out the tortilla chips and have a nice snack while you're waiting to rinse it out.

You will need:

½ ripe avocado (if your hair is long, use a whole avocado)

2 teaspoons olive oil (if your hair is long, use 3 teaspoons)

[1] In a bowl, mash the avocado. Add the oil and mix well.

[2] Apply the mixture to your hair, distributing well from roots to ends. Leave on for 15 minutes or so.

[3] Rinse out and shampoo and condition as usual. Toss the leftovers—they won't keep.

Makes one treatment.

hot oil treatment for extremely
damaged hair

Hot oil is magic. It transforms bland raw potatoes into delicious, glistening French fries. It changes dough into doughnuts. Best of all, it can turn damaged hair into a shiny, shipshape mane. Add herbal essential oils for sweet scents and extra conditioning power. Hot stuff.

You will need:

¼ cup vegetable, olive, coconut, or sweet almond oil, or other oil of your choice (use more oil for long hair)

10 drops essential oil (optional; choose chamomile for light hair, lavender or geranium for normal hair, rosemary for dry or dark hair, lemon or orange for oily hair)

[1] In a glass measuring cup, combine the oils, mixing well.

[2] Microwave the mixture for 20 seconds or so. You want it just warm—not hot hot. Hot oil can cause nasty burns, so be very careful, and have an adult help you.

[3] Apply the mixture to your hair, distributing well from roots to ends. Leave on for 20 minutes.

[4] Rinse out and shampoo and condition as usual.

Makes 2 ounces.

honey

hair gloss

We know—putting sticky stuff in your hair sounds like a really bad idea. If you've ever had to cut a piece of gum out of your locks, you know what we mean. But in small doses, honey does great things for your mane. This polishing rinse gives you shine without stickiness. We think it's the bee's knees.

You will need:

2 cups warm water

¾ teaspoon honey

1 tablespoon lemon juice (optional; best for blondes)

[1] In a pitcher, combine all the ingredients and mix well.

[2] Take the pitcher into the shower with you and shampoo and condition as usual. After you've rinsed out your conditioner, gently wring excess water from your hair, then pour the honey gloss over your head. Don't rinse out. Dry and style as usual.

Makes about 16 ounces.

dewdrop
refresher mist

This spray is like a good night's sleep for your hair; it leaves it looking refreshed and revived. The essential oils condition and make tired locks smell newly shampooed. You'll feel morning-fresh in minutes.

You will need:

Atomizer or spritzer bottle

2 cups water

20 drops essential oil, one type or a mixture (choose chamomile for light hair; rosemary for dark hair; lavender, geranium, or sandalwood for normal hair; carrot or myrrh for dry hair; lemon or tea tree for oily hair)

[1] In the atomizer or spritzer bottle, combine the water and essential oil(s). Shake to mix well.

[2] Spritz the mist on your hair whenever it's looking tired.

Makes 16 ounces.

rich & radiant
color rinses

You don't want a drastic change, and you're deathly afraid of roots. But you want a little more sparkle, a little more spice. These rinses are for you. They subtly bring out your natural highlights. Use more often for more noticeable effects. It's color without commitment, and it looks great on you.

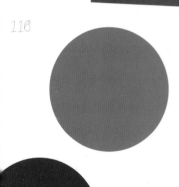

You will need for brunette hair:

2 cups water

2 tea bags (use black tea for brown hair or elderberry tea for black hair)

¼ cup strong coffee

You will need for red hair:

2 cups water

2 red hibiscus tea bags

¼ cup beet or carrot juice, strained

You will need for blonde hair:

2 cups water

2 chamomile tea bags

1 tablespoon lemon juice

[1] In a saucepan, bring the water to a boil. Remove from the heat and add the tea bags. Steep for 15 minutes, then remove the tea bags.

[2] Allow to cool to room temperature. Add the coffee, beet or carrot juice, or lemon juice, whichever you're using.

[3] To use, pour the rinse over your head after you shampoo and condition. You may want to do this over a bowl, so you can catch the runoff and repeat. Leave on for a few minutes, then rinse out.

[4] Dry as usual. Be warned: The rinse can stain clothes and towels, so you'll want to stay away from white until your hair is dry.

Makes one treatment.

sparkle
potion

Anyone can have hair that shines. You want hair that sparkles. This glittery goo does the trick. Slick a little through your 'do and you'll look dazzling all night.

You will need:

½ cup light-hold gel

Fine glitter

Clean, dry container with lid

[1] In a bowl, combine the gel and a healthy sprinkling of glitter. Stir. Add more glitter until you're satisfied with the sparkle level.

[2] To use, work through hair, distributing evenly.

[3] Transfer the remainder to the container and cover tightly for use on your next sparkling occasion.

Makes about 4 ounces.

coconut cream
spritzer

This tropical treat is easy as pie to make. Just blend coconut milk and water for a creamy, dreamy conditioning spray that smells great, too. It's like an island vacation in a bottle. Spritz it on whenever your hair needs a relaxing getaway. It's best for curly locks, as it leaves hair with great curl definition. But go easy on it—a little goes a long way. If you use too much, you may end up with hair that feels more stiff than sassy.

You will need:

2 tablespoons coconut milk

6 tablespoons water

[1] In a spray bottle, combine coconut milk and water. You can change the ratios according to your hair's needs. Use more coconut milk for heavier conditioning, and more water for lighter conditioning. Shake well to mix.

[2] Spray mixture on frizzy, fried locks. Don't wash out.

[3] Store leftover spritzer in the refrigerator. It doesn't have any preservatives, so it can go bad.

Makes 4 ounces.

the end